VISION THERAPY FOR HOME STUDY

A COMPLETE INSTRUCTIONAL BOOK TO IMPROVE FUNCTIONAL VISUAL DEFICIENCIES

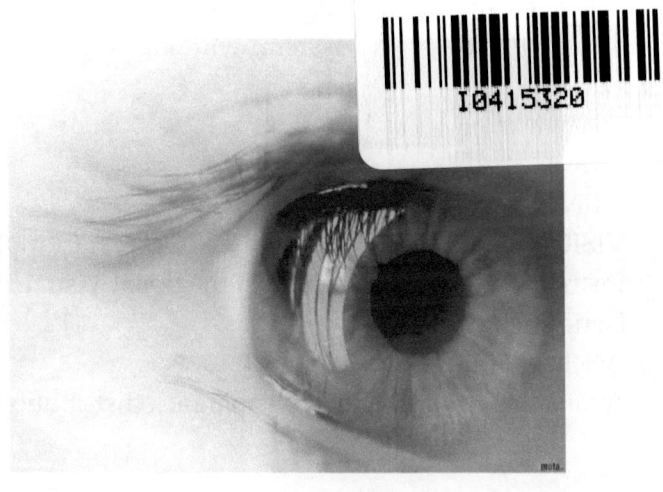

MICHAEL PHILIP GOLDSTEIN, O.D.

ISBN: 978-1-091-09015-6
VISION THERAPY FOR HOME STUDY: A Complete Instructional Book to Improve Functional Visual Deficiencies
 Michael Philip Goldstein, O.D
Available Formats: eBook | Paperback distribution

Acknowledgements

As a child, I suffered from many of the visual symptoms listed in this book. Many years went by without explanation for my Learning problems. Back in the 70's and 80's, we did not have labels of Attention Deficit Disorder, or Attention Deficit Hyperactive Disorder. We were called lazy, learning disabled, or even worse. I would try to do my homework and after a few minutes my eyes were looking at words, but I was not reading. I understood how to read, and what my body needed to do, however, when I looked at the words on a page, my eyes would not track appropriately and would jump around. I saw double often, but since it happened often I thought it was normal. No matter how much I tried, I couldn't control my eyes. It was exhausting, and I would fall asleep when trying to do my homework. I would avoid my homework whenever possible because I knew it would be impossible. Self esteem was low, I couldn't understand what was wrong with me. I felt as if all of my friends could read and do homework much easier than I could, they could take a test and understand what was being asked, I could not.

My personal struggle included special education classes, study skills classes, even trips to school psychologists. The problem is back then we didn't know how important the eyes were to process information we read, and how much impact it had on learning. My parents tried everything they could to help me, hiring extra tutors, study skills teachers, speed reading classes, and even trying to help me create methods to learn information in a way I could understand. IQ testing results showed I scored higher than most, however, my grades did not reflect it.

My personal struggles did not end with me. My parents shared the frustration, and confusion of what the learning problem was. Many long evenings were spent studying with my parents, they helped me learn the material for the upcoming exams. My parents were sure I knew all the information for the test, but when the test was in front of me I could not decipher what they were actually asking. When the test questions had double negatives, it was like reading a foreign language for me.

Years of hard work and dedication allowed me to succeed. Going into Optometry allowed me to learn the visual processes, and not only treat the medical problems people have with their eyes but treat the functional problems that are not always easy to diagnose. In school, I learned the art of vision therapy, and was my own first patient. I would learn techniques in class and go back to my apartment and practice the therapy on myself. I purchased my practice with the goal of treating people with similar problems. My clinic was not only a place for patients to be treated, but also student doctors to learn. Over the years, I've treated thousands of patients with functional vision problems and had exceptional results. It has been my pleasure to help people avoid the struggles that I endured in childhood.

I thank my parents Robert and Gail for all of the sacrifices over the years. They always believed in me, even when I did not believe in myself. In my most difficult days, they were always there to help me and make me a better person. Their support allowed me to acquire a bachelors degree in College and become a doctor in graduate school.

Table of Contents:

1. Introduction
> What is a functional eye disorder, and how does it affect everyday life?
> Refraction and clarity issues
> Tracking issues
> Eye alignment and focusing problems
> Retinal and cortical processing difficulty

2. What is Vision Therapy
> Important pre-therapy questions
> Rules for vision therapy

3. Therapy Sessions
> Weekly half hour sessions
> Sessions listed
> Instructions for therapy exercises
> Tracking exercises
> Circling e's
> Hart Chart
> Post it saccades
> Atari plug and play: Super Breakout with wheel controller
> Ann Arbor Letter Tracking
> Reading with chunking out loud
> Saccadic arrows

Eye Alignment/ Vergence exercises
Red/green or red/blue exercises
Red/green tranaglyph slide
Lifesaver card
Needle and straw
Brock string
Stereograms

4. Definitions

Chapter 1
Introduction

Our eyes are said to be the jewel of the body, according to Henry David Thoreau. I agree that the eyes are important for beauty, but the function of the organ is truly impressive.

Our sight is one of the 5 major senses we use to survive. Hearing, touch, smell, taste, and sight help us move in our world, know what is good and bad, learn, and protect us from danger. Our senses can change our mood, they can make you happy or sad, relaxed or create anxiety.

As children, our learning is 80 % by vision. We look at our teachers, we read books, we study our written notes. Our eyes need to perceptually identify what we are seeing, track objects, and team (align). We need to make sure what we are seeing is clear by flexing our lens in the eye and controlling when to flex and relax the muscle.

Are the images we are seeing being accurately transmitted and processed by our brain? The electric signal from the eye to the optic nerve must travel throughout the brain until it gets to the occipital cortex (the back of the brain). The occipital cortex puts together the electric code to create the "vision" of what our target was.

A functional eye disorder is when a piece of this process is not working correctly, and this gives the <u>same symptoms as a learning disability, dyslexia, or attention deficit disorder.</u>

Are you or any family members experiencing any of these issues? If a person suffers from this kind of problem, symptoms could demonstrate as: blurred vision, difficulty tracking, trouble understanding what is being read, being a slow reader, excessive time spent on homework, difficulty between sight and motor coordination, vertigo, headaches, double vision, mixing up words, avoidance of near tasks such as reading, frustration and acting out.

If any of these symptoms sound familiar, it is important to have a comprehensive eye examination with an optometrist or ophthalmologist that is familiar with these functional eye problems and are able to rule out medical health issues. Normally, a doctor will have the title of Behavioral Optometrist or Developmental Optometrist. To find a doctor in your area, the American Optometric Association or College of Optometrists in Visual Development can help. A comprehensive eye examination can rule out other dangerous medical problems which can give the same symptoms as a functional eye disorder.

When learning is obstructed, or difficult, we need to examine the eyes to make sure they are not the cause, since they are a major piece of learning. We are very lucky to have symptoms as red flags if vision is not working correctly. Headaches (usually in the forehead) are common, losing place when reading, double vision, vertigo, avoidance of near tasks, poor coordination, slow reading, are a few of the complaints one might have.

This book will serve as an aid for our population of "<u>vision related learning disabilities</u>" or people suffering from <u>functional vision problems</u>. Hopefully, you will have the same success we have had in my clinic in Rocky Hill Connecticut over the years. The training program listed in this book will only work with motivation and repetition. Results may vary depending on the problem and person and results cannot be guaranteed.

What is a functional eye disorder, and how does it affect everyday life?

Before I answer this, we need to discuss the basics on how the visual system works. Let's create a process for vision from the beginning to end.

First, a target is needed. The target could be any object that is large enough to be seen by the human eye. Let us say our target for discussion is a penny. Once we have a target in mind, we need to aim our eye at it to allow the light reflecting off the object to enter into the eye. We have two major focusing pieces of tissue, the cornea and the lens. The cornea is the very front of the eye, a clear piece of tissue that covers the iris and pupil. Once light focuses through the cornea, it travels through the anterior segment of the eye through the hole in the iris called the pupil. At this point, the lens bends the light again before traveling through the posterior segment towards the retina. The sensory retina is the tissue which senses the light from the target and uses intricate signals to create the image of the object to be sent through the optic nerve towards the occipital lobe of the brain.

The first possible functional eye problem could be difficulty aiming the eye at the target. Especially, if the target is moving. If the target is moving slowly and smoothly the eye tracking is called a pursuit movement. If the target is moving in quick bursts the eye tracking is named saccadic eye movements. To make the process a little more difficult, we have two eyes we need to align. We will discuss ocular alignment problems in the chapters to follow.

The next functional problem would be an image that is not in focus. This means the cornea might not be bending the light appropriately to focus on the retina. If the light is focusing before the retina this is called nearsightedness or myopia. Refractive correction might be necessary to focus the light to the retina (spectacles, contact lenses, refractive surgery). If the light is bending and focusing behind the retina, this is called farsightedness or hyperopia. This is when the second refracting part of the eye comes into use, the lens. As the lens flexes, the image of the target moves forward towards the retina, and ultimately can be focused on it. When the lens flexes, it is the same as flexing any muscle in the body. It can become fatigued or sore with heavy use.

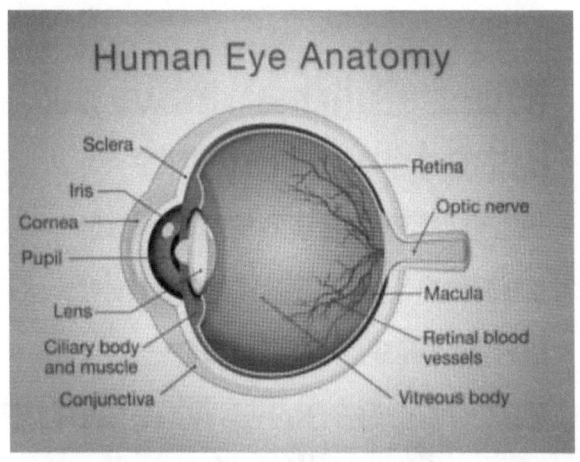

Anatomy of the eye

Again, refractive correction (glasses, contacts, etc) can focus the light to the retina to relax the lens. Once the image is in focus, the retina needs to process the information you are looking at. The retina becomes stimulated by the light and sends the information to the optic nerve. Once we are finished viewing our target, our eyes move to look at something else. In order to see the next image, our retina must "mask" (erase) the image from the first object. Some people have difficulty erasing the image burned into the retinal cells, and this can lead to confusion when trying to see the next image. Think about a chalk board, if a word is written and not erased well. It will be very difficult to recognize the next word written on top of the preceding one. This can create problems with reading. This is a masking problem.

Most children have no
idea how they are
supposed to see. So
when words look like
this, they assume
everyone sees the same
way they do. Imagine
how frustrating that
would be.

Example of Masking problems

Refraction and clarity issues:

A comprehensive eye examination can include the determination for prescriptive lenses. If a person has blurry vision they might be nearsighted or farsighted, have astigmatism, an eye disease, or amblyopia. When we discussed nearsightedness and farsightedness on the previous page, however astigmatism is slightly more complicated.

Astigmatism is when the cornea is not shaped like a sphere cut in half. When the cornea is shaped like a half sphere, all the light passing through it focuses at the same point no matter which meridian. Now, picture a football, where you have one long flat meridian, and one steep short meridian. Light passing through those different curvatures will focus in different places. The steeper meridian will bend light more, and make that focus point closer to the front of the eye. The flatter meridian will bend light less and focus light posterior, or further from the front of the eye. Corrective lenses or refractive surgery can correct for this difference in focusing, and focus all the light in a single spot. The difference in curvature (astigmatism) can be mild or significant. When significant, this can create a constant blurry vision if not discovered early, and can even impact visual development. If the brain does not get a clear signal from the retina in the blurry meridian, it might not develop in that meridian in order to appreciate a clear image. This is called meridional amblyopia.

If a person has significant farsightedness (hyperopia), the brain has multiple choices. First, it might decide to leave the vision blurry, and not try to clear the image by focusing the crystalline lens. This can cause refractive amblyopia, meaning the brain does not learn to see clearly in all meridians in each eye because the image to the retina is constantly blurry. Without a clear picture the brain will not learn to see a clear picture. If the brain chooses to focus the crystalline lens (to move the focus point forward to the retina), making the image clear in one eye, this can cause an eye turn called Accommodative Esotropia.

The harder you focus the lens in your eye, the more the eyes will turn in towards your nose. This can also be called Strabismus. With an eye turn such as this, if the brain chooses to turn one eye constantly, this can cause amblyopia (delayed development in the brain from not having a clear image or suppressing the eye) in the turned eye, and the person can develop clear sight through the straight eye only. If the eye turn is alternating, this gives a better chance the person can see out of both eyes sufficiently. However, an alternating eye turn (alternating esotropia) can become a constant eye turn (constant esotropia) if left untreated. This is a person that needs the farsighted prescription glasses as early as possible to deter refractive or strabismic amblyopia. They would also need active patching or vision therapy techniques.

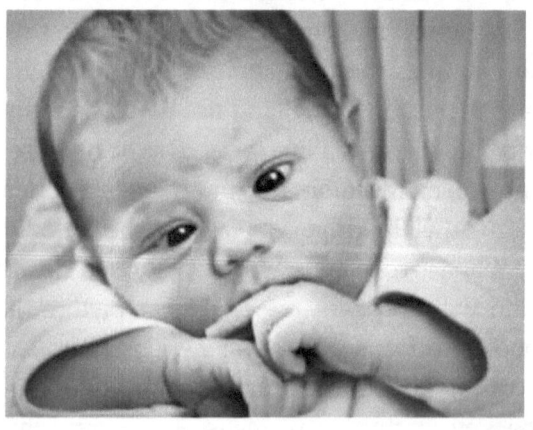

Example of Esotropia

A nearsighted or myopic person is much less likely to have amblyopia, because when they look at near objects they are able to see a clear image that the brain can process and develop. However, they have a distance blur which spectacles would be needed to clear. A problem can arise from a person who has one nearsighted eye, and one farsighted eye and no spectacle correction. Depending on the prescription, if the person cannot make both eyes clear at the same time, they might choose one eye to see, and the other to shut off. The brain will always select the easier eye to see with. This can also create a refractive amblyopia.

The important thing to know, is the earlier a refractive issue is discovered, and corrected, the less likely to have amblyopia and permanent vision loss. The recommendation of the American Optometric Association is a 6 month old well visit exam, followed by a 5-6 year old exam before the child begins school. After the age of 6, a yearly Eye exam should be performed by an optometrist or ophthalmologist.

Tracking issues:

Tracking problems are usually detected with a person having poor coordination, or appearing clumsy. In school, this issue can manifest by difficulty keeping place when reading, or trouble having clear writing with difficulty spacing letters and words.

It's extremely common for people to complain of losing place when reading, or having to re-read the same sentence multiple times to comprehend. Schools tend to use straight edges or rulers to teach kids to track better, however, they are learning to compensate with a device. This does not fix the problem, it merely makes them depended on the device. It is understandable why schools do this, they are not there to fix this problem, they are there to teach information. The schools have such high demand these days to pump the kids full of information. The basic skills that were learned years ago may become overlooked. Appropriate tracking abilities can be taught at any age using therapy, without the need from supportive devices.

As mentioned earlier, we have pursuit eye movements (smooth tracking) and saccadic eye movements (quick jumping motions). Both are used in efficient reading. In order to efficiently use these eye movements, we also need to understand the "global search mechanism".

When we are young, we learn to read by scanning each letter in every word. This is how we sound out the word. But as we age, our system changes. We begin to identify the words by their shape. As an older child or adult, we can even read a whole sentence without one letter, just by drawing the shapes of the words next to each other. This is how we are able to read with a smooth flow. When we are looking at one word, our peripheral vision (side vision) notices the shape of the words next to it and puts it together in an information chunk. We should not be reading one word at a time for fluency, we should be reading 3-4 words in a chunk based on what we are seeing.

Try to read this:

Example 1

Theboyandhisdogwenttothestore.whileatthestoret heboypurchasedgumandothertreats.whenhegothome hehadabellyache.

Without proper spacing of the words, we cannot identify the shapes, and this shuts down our global search mechanism.

Example 2

The boy and his dog went to the store. While at the store the boy purchased gum and other treats. When he got home he had a belly ache.

As you can see, it is much easier to read example 2 when the global search mechanism is utilized. Imagine if a person does not learn this chunking ability, that would be the student in Example 1.

Eye alignment and focusing problems:

Once we have a target in sight, our eyes must align to see the target at the same time. When each eye is aimed at the same object at a slightly different angle, this very small change is what gives us depth perception and stereopsis (3D vision). Other ways we compensate to recognize distances is by object size, color, clarity, etc. If both eyes are not aimed at the target, the brain will either see double or suppress (shut off) an eye. An eye alignment problem may be intermittent and not constant. So when a person fatigues the eye might turn inward or outward. A common intermittent eye alignment problem is called convergence insufficiency. This is when someone has difficulty turning the eyes inward towards the nose to see a near object.

This problem is the most common eye alignment problem, with an estimated twenty percent of the population suffering. Someone may complain of double or blurry vision when trying to read. This can also affect coordination and balance.

Imagine a line drawn from the middle of your forehead all the way to the floor. This line separates the right side of your body from the left. Most people during development have trouble crossing their midline. This means using the right hand on the left side of your body and left hand on the right side of the body. The same is common with convergence insufficiency. When we read in the United States we read left to right on a page. If your eyes are not lining up correctly, and if you are shutting off an eye, the suppressed eye will alternate based on where you are looking. So if we start reading on the left, the left eye will turn on (and the right eye will shut off and drift outward). When we get to the middle of the page, now the right eye needs to turn on (and the left will shut off and drift outward). Jumping between the eyes like this when reading will cause the words to appear to move when reading, or make it very difficult to keep your place. Some people do not shut off the misaligned eye, and they complain of double vision when reading.

Another subconscious technique for our brain to compensate, is to focus the crystalline lens excessively. When the lens focuses, it also sends a signal to our brain saying we are looking up close. Usually, when we look at near objects out eyes turn inward and we focus in a proper ratio. But if the eyes are not turning in enough, we can focus harder and the eyes can be forced to turn inward. This extreme over focusing can cause major fatigue, and normally people cannot read more than 15 minutes before they get a headache or fall asleep from the over exertion. Some eye doctors out there might give you reading glasses for this problem, but that only takes away your only method to try and line up the eyes by relaxing your focusing with the lens. Without that over focusing the eyes are not aligned. If someone is using the over focusing to line up their eyes at near, this can also cause a person to appear more nearsighted than they really are. If that lens is focusing really hard it may be difficult to relax it after looking up close. This accommodative (focusing) spasm can make your distance vision blurry if it does not relax, and sometimes these people can be prescribed distance glasses when they don't really need them.

Convergence insufficiency is extremely responsive to vision therapy and can be fixed in the matter of months.

Problems with eye alignment don't only happen with near tasks, they can also occur when viewing objects in the distance. People can have Exotropia (when an eye turns outward towards the ear), or Esotropia (when the eye turns inward towards the nose). People with congenital exotropia (born with it) generally have good vision in both eyes, but the brain alternates between the two eyes. Congenital esotropia (born with it) can alternate between the two eyes which has a better visual prognosis than a constant esotropia (the same eye is always turned).

Retinal and cortical processing difficulty

As discussed earlier, the focused image is projected onto the retina to stimulate the retinal cells. Once these cells are stimulated, we have to be efficient in erasing the image to make way for the next image. Masking ability can be reduced due to the lens over focusing the eye.

When the crystalline lens over focuses to try and correct for alignment problems, or correct for farsightedness, it also makes the light focusing into the eye have more contrast. The increased contrast happens when someone over focuses. This will create black to appear darker, and white to appear lighter. When that high contrast is stimulating the retinal cells, they also have to work harder. So, if we can help the lens relax, it should help with masking issues. Many schools are using Irlen transparent colored overlays to try and reduce the contrast of print on a book. The only colors that can reduce the contrast are blue and green (cool colors). Red, yellow, and other warm colors will stimulate the crystalline lens to accommodate (focus) more and make the print have more contrast, ultimately increasing contrast making masking more difficult. Again, the Irlen transparent lens is a compensatory tool, but will not fix the problem.

Chapter 2
What is Vision Therapy?

Now that we have a basic understanding of all these components of vision, let's discuss the goal of vision therapy. We understand we have three major parts to vision, tracking, eye alignment, and focusing (accommodation). Think of these three components linked together in a triad, and if one piece doesn't work well, the other two might try to over compensate. When training the eyes, it is important to target the component of the triad that needs to be trained. At the beginning it is better to train each component separately, then as the weeks progress, try to meld them back together. In order to separate these components, we will use reading glasses, eye patches, and sometimes red/ green or red/ blue filtered eyeglasses. Since this is an instructional book on home therapy we are going to use everyday tools you may have around the house. Charts and tools can be self created or purchased on the internet.

Of course an in office therapy program will have more resources, but we can still achieve the same results with alternative therapy.

In my private practice I've had the pleasure of providing vision therapy for thousands of people, and even trained graduating Optometrists from different Optometry Schools. The program I'm sharing in this book is the same basic program I used in my practice for the past 18 years. Normally, patients would finish the therapy program in 3 months with a once per week office visit, and home therapy exercises for 10-15 minutes per day.

This program is a generalization of techniques and exercises, and the goal of this book is to provide a standardized template for people to follow. These programs should give successful results for vision related learning problems as mentioned previously. Remember, it is very important to have a comprehensive eye examination to check the overall health of the eye, and this book does not replace a thorough exam.

Important pre-therapy questions:

1. Do you see double?

20 percent of the human population suffer from Convergence Insufficiency. This is when it is difficult to turn the eyes inwards towards your nose in order to look at near objects. In my practice, I hear children say "yes" often when asked if they see double. They don't realize they are not supposed to because it has always been there. It feels normal for them. Many parents don't believe their child, because it is difficult to think that all these years they never knew. If you ask the child they will tell you.

2. Do you get headaches?

This is the most common complaint with people coming into my office. Usually, they are located in the middle of the forehead, and they can feel relief when they press on the sore spot, or close their eyes. If the person presses on the sore area and it hurts more, this is usually a sign of sinus problems. Headaches from functional eye problems usually occur after 10-15 minutes of near work. This includes computer, reading, tablet computers, and playing on phones.

3. Does it feel like your vision fluctuates? Does your vision feel blurred in the distance after doing near tasks?

Again, the crystalline lens in the eye is needed to focus a little at near, and relax in the distance. It's sole responsibility is to focus light onto the retina to be clear. However, if it is working very hard to keep the eyes aligned, the lens can spasm. Once the lens is spasming, this can cause the distance vision to become blurred because the lens is having trouble relaxing the way it should to look far away. A common complaint is "I have trouble driving home at night after work because my vision is very blurry. But when I am not working, I don't notice the blurry vision throughout the day".

4. Do words move around on the page when you are reading? Are you a slow reader?

We have a skill where we can cross our midline of our body, using the right parts on the left side, and the left parts on the right side. This is called crossing our midline. It sounds very simple, but it is a very complex neurological process. Different sides of our brain control different sides of our body. Our right side of the brain controls the left side of the body under the neck, and the left side of the brain controls the right side of our body under the neck.

When we read, we begin on the left side of the page, cross over the midline and finish reading on the right side of the page. After we are finished with that line, we cross back to the left side of the page again. To add difficulty, if the eyes are not teaming together, then we might be using the left eye to read on the left side of the page (and suppress the right eye), and when we cross over to the right side of the page passed the midline, we switch to the right eye (and suppress the left). The constant switching between the eyes at the midline will cause the words to jump, or swim on the paper.

5. Does it take you longer to complete homework, or other tasks than others?

It makes sense if you are working so hard to compensate for the functional problem it will take more concentration and more time. Think about when you are driving a car, when you are in familiar territory you might have the radio blaring and can be multitasking mentally. But when you get close to your destination in an unfamiliar area, how often do we turn down the radio, or turn it off completely? We can no longer multitask mentally, and need to give navigation our full attention.

6. Do you suffer from poor written test scores even though you know the material when studying?

As mentioned before, it is a long process to acquire the information you are looking at, process it, and then respond with motor movement. If the process is interrupted, it can also make us misunderstand what we are being asked. You might feel you are answering the question perfectly, however, there may be an extra word (such as not, won't, can't), or a double negative that makes it almost impossible for you to understand the question. You may not see part of the sentence and answer the opposite of what is intended.

7. Have you been told you have attention issues?

I can guarantee if you have a functional vision disorder, it will appear you have ADD, ADHD, or a learning disability. It is difficult, sometimes is even painful to try and perform a task through all of these obstacles. If someone is given the choice to read a book that is double, and gives them headaches; or get up and talk to you friends, that is an easy choice for many people.

8. Do you have low self esteem?

The person who is affected by a vision related learning disability does not understand why things are so hard for them. Everyone around them must be smarter because they read faster, get better grades, can pay attention better, and may not study as much. Actually, most people suffering with the vision related learning disabilities work harder, have stronger stamina, and can be smarter than people who don't work as hard. They find ways to compensate for their deficiency by trying to puzzle solve, and many times are very successful. These are the people who are among the brightest, but will say they are not good test takers. These are the people who when get out into the work force, go to work early, and usually stay late.

Rules for vision therapy:

It is extremely important to follow certain rules when performing therapy. If the rules are not followed you may not see improvement, and sometimes can even reinforce bad habits which will make your eyes worse. Please keep the below rules in mind when doing the exercises.

1. When reading, use "Harmon's Distance". This is the length measured from a person's knuckles to the elbow. This number will change based on the size of the person. Most adults are approximately 16", while children are closer to 12". This is the distance a person should have their face away from the reading material or near task.
2. Whenever doing a tracking task, the person should not move their head. Only eye movements are allowed during tracking. If the persons head moves during the exercise, they might not notice. So if someone is observing, a gentle reminder is important to correct the movement.
3. If training convergence or other eye alignment problems, no eye patch is needed.
4. If you are training focusing (accommodation), you can separate from eye alignment exercises, and train only focusing by using an eye patch.

5. When reading, a finger or other tools should not be used. This goes with all tracking exercises. Only use your eyes for eye tracking and reading during therapy. When improvement is made, discontinue tracking tools from real life as well.

6. Repetition is very important. A half hour vision therapy session once a week will teach the skill and measure improvement. Daily therapy training sessions will reinforce the skill.

7. At the beginning, everything will be difficult for the person undergoing therapy. That is why therapy is needed, if therapy is easy they would not need it. Keep at it! The first few sessions we expect poor results, make sure all scores are recorded. This will be used as your baseline measurements. From those scores you will keep track of improvement.

8. Ibuprofen may be indicated if you are cleared by your primary physician for the first two half hour sessions. The therapy can create headaches if the eyes are not functioning correctly, and you are learning the correct way.

9. Any success is still a success. If working with a child, make a big deal when they can do something new, or get a higher score than before. Positive reinforcement will make them motivated. They also like knowing they are learning secrets that not everyone knows to

make their eyes work better. These secrets will also make them a better reader in school, better at sports, etc.

10. Chunk information whenever possible. Try not to read one letter or word at a time. Every exercise should involve two to three letters or words to teach chunking and better use of peripheral vision (global search mechanism).

11. Learn the reading rhythm. Reading should sound beautiful, like a song or poem. Not like a robot.

Chapter 3
Therapy exercises

Weekly half hour session:

Once per week, there should be a half hour therapy session. This is the session which you begin a new daily homework program. Each half hour session should consist of two exercises. You will have the exercises pre-programmed in this book. Again, you will train each of the three components (tracking, eye alignment, and focusing) independently, and then add them back together as the weeks go on.

The daily homework assignments will only be one exercise, and should be approximately 10-15 minutes per day.

You will need to get some inexpensive supplies from the pharmacy. You will need +1.00 reading glasses if you do not currently have an eyeglass prescription. If you wear contact lenses you can still use the reading glass mentioned if you are under 40 years old. If you wear eyeglasses full time, and you are under 40, you can order eyeglass reading clip on's through the internet for training (these clip right to your normal spectacle frame). If you currently wear some sort of bifocal or progressive eyeglass you do not need anything else.

You will also need an eye patch (the best are the ones with an elastic band). Below, I will list the therapy sessions, the exercises, and the daily therapy routine (the exercise you will practice every day) for the week.

Session 1:

1. Circling e's with eye patch. Circle for 10 minutes, then switch patch to opposite eye and correct. Please see instructions for "circling e's".
2. Hart Chart with one eye patched. Please see instructions for "Hart Chart Monocular"

Daily homework should be circling e's the same way as during session 1.

Session 2:

1. Hart Chart monocular or with one eye patched. Please see instructions for "Hart Chart Monocular".
2. BI Stereograms for 15 minutes. Please follow instructions for "BI Stereograms".

Daily homework Hart Chart once per eye each day the same as in session 2.

Session 3:

1. BI Stereograms for 15 minutes. Please follow instructions for "BI Stereograms".
2. Brock String for 10 minutes. Please follow instructions for "Brock String".

Daily homework BI Stereograms as performed in session 3.

Session 4:

1. Brock String for 10 minutes. Please follow instructions for "Brock String".
2. Post it saccades standing on one foot. Please see instructions for "Post it saccades".

Daily homework Brock String for 10 minutes per day as performed in session 4.

Session 5:

1. Post it saccades standing on one foot. Please see instructions for "Post it saccades".
2. BO Lifesaver Card for 15 minutes. Please see instructions for " BO Lifesaver Card".

Daily homework Post it saccades. Please perform as you did in session 5.

Session 6:

1. BO Lifesaver Card for 15 minutes. Please see instructions for " BO Lifesaver Card"
2. BO Stereograms for 15 minutes. Please see instructions for "BO Stereograms".

Daily homework BO Lifesaver card. Perform as you did in session 6.

Session 7:

1. BO Stereograms for 15 minutes. Please see instructions for "BO Stereograms".
2. Reading with Chunking 15 minutes. Please see instructions for Reading with Chunking".

Daily homework BO Stereograms. Perform as you did in session 7.

Session 8:

1. Reading with Chunking. Please follow instructions for "Reading with Chunking".
2. BI Lifesaver card. Please follow instructions for "BI Lifesaver card".

Daily homework Reading with Chunking. Perform as you did in session 8.

Session 9:

1. BI Lifesaver Card. Please follow instructions for BI Lifesaver card.
2. Jump BI and BO Lifesaver card. Please follow instructions for BI and BO Jump Lifesaver card.

Daily homework BI Lifesaver Card. Perform as you did in session 9.

Session 10:

1. Jump BI and BO Lifesaver card. Please follow instructions for BI and BO Lifesaver card.
2. Jump BI and BO Stereograms. Please follow instructions for BI and BO Stereograms.

Daily homework Jump BI and BO Stereograms. Perform as you did in session 10.

Session 11:

1. Jump BI and BO Stereograms. Please follow instructions for BI and BO Stereograms.
2. Circling e's binocular. Please follow instructions for circling e's binocular.

Daily homework Jump BI and BO Stereograms. Perform as you did in session 11.

Session 12:

1. Circling e's binocular. Please follow instructions for circling e's binocular.
2. Reading with Chunking. Please follow instructions for Reading with Chunking.

Instructions for exercises

Please note not all of the exercises listed are in this program, however you can do extra exercises to add to the core therapy routine.

Tracking exercises:

Circling e's (can be monocular, one eye; or binocular, 2 eyes)

1. Place the patch over one eye. You should be using +1.00 reading glasses, or +1.00 reading clip-on over your glasses.
2. Find a magazine article with black print on a white background. This print should be regular sized magazine print.
3. Search for e's with one eye covered, and not using the pen or finger to search. After an "e" is located, now you can move the hand to the paper to circle the letter. After the "e" is

circled, you must move the hand off the paper as if it were hot.

4. When searching for e's, make sure you scan from left to right, one line at a time, as if you are reading. However, you do not need to read the words, just searching for letters.

5. Circle the "e's" left to right line by line for 10 minutes. We chose the letter "e" since it is the most common letter in print.

6. After you are finished circling, return to the top of the paragraph where you began, and correct. To correct, you will patch the opposite eye. At this point you can use a straight edge to underline the line only when correcting, but still do not use a pen or finger to keep place. When you see an "e" that you missed, cross it out with an "X".

After correcting the assignment, count how many "x's" you wrote on the paper. This is your score, the lower the number of "x's" the better the score. It should be recorded as number of x's(right eye or left eye) depending on which eye you circled with. So 15xR means 15 e's were missed when circling with your right eye and correcting with your left. Every day, you should switch to the opposite eye when circling. If circled with the right eye yesterday, circle with the left today (and correct with the right).

Hart Chart: (you should be able to find on the internet, or create your own)

Should always be one eye at a time, monocular. Please see the two charts labeled Hart Chart.

1. Hold the small chart in you hand and have the large chart on the wall in front of you about eye level. You should be approximately 5 feet from the wall.
2. Read the letters out loud on the first line of the small chart in your hand. Make sure you "chunk" the information by two or three letters at a time. Groups of two are good for very young kids, three's are good for older kids and adults.
3. After reading the first line on the chart in your hand, then read the first line on the wall the same way while chunking out loud.
4. Next read the second line on the chart in your hand the same way. Then switch to the second line on the chart on the wall.
5. Repeat to the next line, etc. after you finish the distance and near chart, repeat the process with the opposite eye.

Please see examples of Hart Chart below:

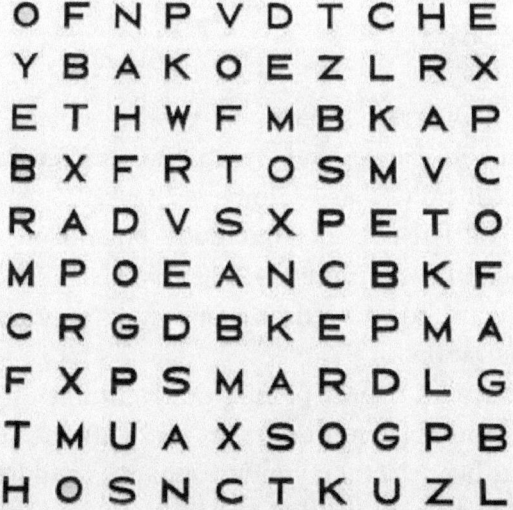

Large Hart Chart

```
Y L 4 B E A 8 U M H
K 2 D S U 4 L O F Z
H C 7 A E T 3 1 Y R
P B 9 G N O 5 R V T
L 2 K G B 5 U T 3 D
A W E S 8 R O X N 1
7 A P T 6 E N U R Z
V 4 R 9 S M X 2 J T
S O 2 N 6 E H U 5 W
L 8 V S P D 1 N G 7
```

Small Hart Chart

Post it saccades:

Standing on one foot balancing or standing on balance board.

1. On dry erase board or post it notes. Write numbers 1 through 10 with one number on each post it note. Place numbers 2,4,6,8,10 vertically on the left side of your body but not in order. Place the odd numbers 1,3,5,7,9 on the right side of your body vertically and not in order. See illustration.
2. Point with a laser pointer or bright flash light to each number in order from 1-10 without moving your head. You may move your eyes and hand in order to aim the light. You should point to a number on the left, then switch to a number on the right, then left, etc. if the head moves, sometimes we don't notice it, so it is good to have an observer watching to help you correct. If the head moves, or if balancing on one foot and the other foot touches the ground, you must begin again from number one. If on a balance board, start over if the edge of the balance board touches the floor from loss of balance.
3. If you begin to memorize the order of the numbers you can rearrange them, still with evens on one side and odds on the other. If standing on one foot, alternate feet with each cycle.
4. It is important to go slow, with pointing at least one number per second, do not go faster than

that. This exercise should go about 10 minutes with alternating feet.

5. If standing on balance board during this exercise, to make the task more challenging, move feet outward from center of board towards the edges for more distribution of weight.

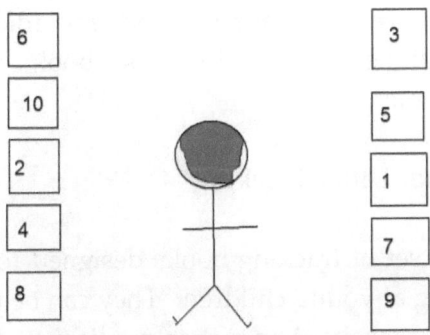

Post it Saccade illustration

Atari Plug and Play: Superbreakout with wheel controller

Can be purchased online through amazon or find a retro gaming store, excellent eye hand tracking exercise.

1. This exercise works on eye hand coordination, tracking, and passing midline, and fine motor coordination.

2. When tracking the ball on the screen, make sure the person playing is centered within the screen,

and is not moving their head, just tracking with their eyes.

3. Record the score after each game, this is how you will measure improvement with the fine motor and tracking control.

4. As the person gets better at this game, there is a setting where you can play 2 balls at the same time. This will switch your tracking from pursuit movements to pursuit and saccadic tracking (mentioned early in this book with eye movements).

Ann Arbor Letter Tracking

This is a set of tracking books designed for all ages, beginning at young children. They can be purchased from the website Ann Arbor publishers. It is easily searchable online as well.

1. Each paragraph is one cycle through the exercise. The goal is for you to circle the letters of the alphabet in order without skipping any. If you skip a letter, you will not be able to get to "Z". When doing this exercise, you should have one eye covered with the eye patch, and when doing a different paragraph switch the patch to the opposite eye.

2. Search with your eyes, do not use a pen or finger to search for the letters. Once you see the letter you are searching for, you may circle it, but then

move your hand away promptly and resume eye tracking. Remember, Harmon's Distance!

3. Time how long it takes to do a paragraph, and write it down. Depending on how long it takes to do a paragraph, you can either do one paragraph or page per night for homework. There are different levels of books. Large print for younger kids, to small print for older people.

ABCDEFGHIJKLMNOPQRSTUVWXYZ
a b c d e f g h i j k l m n o p q r s t u v w x y z

Hoft arn holby kelm croe peurot. Ix rish. Dop fult hurs lim kreph thoz tfol krik nul guar quim. Auth quat rulk tay suild meve neb poj durat. Ceth boft kalb non rem turz bured dir ench verf thay. Forg chat apite. Bague quide tere gusk malf bache deph left Wald mund newk pov fam wemp snal fron. Mex jop yonde baza

___ Min. ___ Sec.

Arom bixto. Heen dolk roche hekis

Example of Ann Arbor Letter Tracing

Reading with chunking out loud:

1. First, record yourself reading without any sort of correction.
2. Then give tips:
    A) Read 2-3 words at a time (chunk)
    B) Obey punctuation! At a period, count to 2. At a comma, count to one. At an exclamation point, raise your voice or shout, etc. many people read like a robot and don't use punctuation correctly.

3. After you practice this, get the rhythm of two to three words at a time, make your voice go up and down. Break the robot reading! Make sure when you read it sounds like a poem or song.
4. Then, record yourself with all the new tips. Listen to the difference. It may take many tries to get this to sound natural, keep at it.

Saccadic arrows:

Create a document with rows of arrows randomly pointing up, down, left, and right. The arrows should be large enough to have approximately 9-12 arrows per line. You can draw them by hand or type them with computer at a larger font. You should have about 15 lines of random arrows.

1.Hang the arrow chart on the wall approximately 6 feet in front of you.

2. Track the arrows left to right as if reading, and say the direction of the arrows out loud. Make sure you verbally "chunk" the arrows (say two or three directions at a time). Ex. Up-down-left, in one breath. Go rhythmically like reading and chunking.
3. If you make a mistake, begin at the beginning of that line and repeat.
See example below:

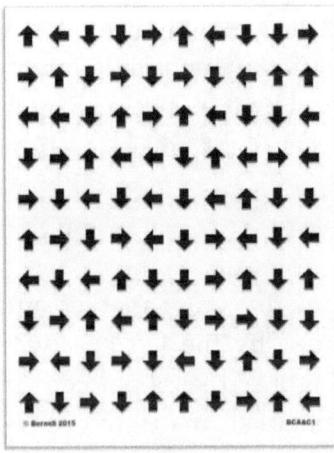

Example of Saccadic Arrow Chart

Eye alignment/ Vergence exercises:

Red/green or red/blue exercises:

Red/green vergence exercises will work on eye alignment. Red/green or red/blue training glasses may be difficult to get, but if you can find them they are very valuable. You can search for these online. They can also avoid suppression of an eye. When wearing red/green or red/blue glasses, always place the red lens over the right eye.

On therapy exercises utilizing red/green filters, there will be a red image and a green image. When the images separate they can cause your eyes to converge or diverge (turn inward or outward). The red image is seen by the eye using the green lens when looking at a pigmented image like ink. And the red lens will see the green pigmented image.

However, this is the opposite if you are looking at colored lights. Red light will be seen by the eye in the red lens, and green light will be seen by the eye in the green lens.

Example: a red dry erase marker on a dry erase board will be seen by the left eye (with the green lens). But if using a red laser pointer to point at the image from the marker, the right eye (red lens) will see the laser light.

Red/green tranaglyph slide (bunny, clown, faces, airplane) (again, you can search for these online)

Pigmented red and green target. So left eye see's red picture and right eye see's green picture.

When you separate the images where the red picture moves to the right and the green image moves to the left, this makes your eyes converge (cross inward) to see one image. You should hold the single image as long as you can while moving the slides slowly. When the picture becomes blurry, this is the brains way of telling you you are about to lose the fusion of the image. If the image becomes blurry stop moving the slide, and stare at the picture until the image becomes clear again. Once clear again, move the slides apart again until the image becomes blurry or double. When the image becomes double, the arrow at the bottom of the slide will point at the score. Record that value. With convergence, the optical illusion of the image will appear smaller and closer.

Likewise, if the images separate with the green slide moving to the right and the red moving to the left, this will cause the eyes to to turn outward or diverge. With divergence, the image will look larger and further away.

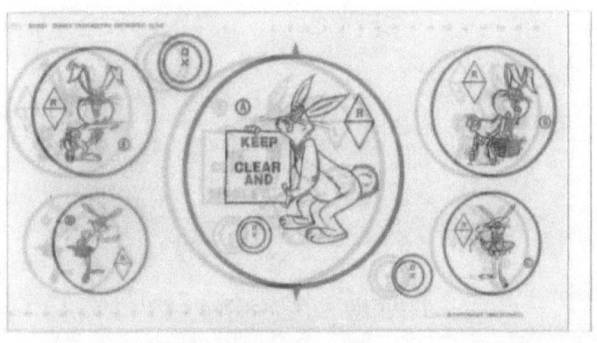

Example of Red Green Bunny Tranaglyph

Non red/green vergence training techniques:

Lifesaver card: you can find online or create your own

Translucent or opaque cards are available. Translucent is good for helping someone learn divergence, because they can look through the card to turn their eyes outward. Opaque makes divergence more difficult, but helps with convergence.

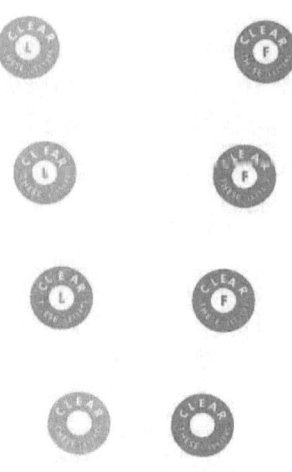

Example of Lifesaver Card

BO Lifesaver card: you can search online or create your own

Wear +1.00 reading glasses or +1.00 clip on over your glasses if under 40 years old.

> 1. Hold lifesaver card 16-18 inches away.
> 2. Place pencil tip or pointer directly between the two circles on the bottom line. The bottom line is the set of circles that are closest together. Slowly move the pointer closer to your eyes while staring at the pointer. At the moment you see three circles behind the pointer instead of two, this gives us the fusion we are looking for. Hold the three circles for 5 seconds.
> 3. Then move to the next line of circles above. Repeat the process.

Once you get good at fusing the image with the pointer to make three circles on each line, try to do it without the pointer (just by crossing your eyes).

BI Lifesaver card:

> 1. Hold the card 16-18 inches away.
> 2. Look past the card at a distance object. Slowly move the card into your line of sight without looking directly at the card. Notice the bottom line of circles. Your eyes will be aligned at a further distance (past the card).

3. Stare through the card until the two circles become three.

4. Repeat the process with the next line above the one you just did.   Hold fusion for 5 seconds.

Needle and Straw:

1. Have someone hold a drinking straw vertically and directly in front of you. Start with the distance approximately 16" away from your nose.

2. You should be holding a straightened paperclip vertically at the very top. You should not feel for the hole, but should use your depth perception to locate the distance. If you miss on a try, move your hand away and try again.If the eyes are not aligned, you will see multiple straws.

3. Try to place the straightened paper clip into the vertical straw.

4. With each insertion of the paper clip into the straw, remove the clip, and have the other person slowly move the straw close to make you converge more.

Brock String: Can find online, or even create your own from a craft store. Need beads and a long string.

1. Tie one end to a door knob, or stable object.

2. Hold the opposite end to the middle of your nose.

3. Space the beads out evenly, with the distance bead all the way to the far end of the string, and the closest bead to your nose about 12" away.

4. Look at the near bead. The bead you are looking at should be single, and all others should appear double. Likewise, the string should cross exactly at the bead you are looking at. When done correctly, the two strings will be visible and double beads should appear where ever you are not looking.

5. Stare at the bead for 5 seconds.

6. Then move your fixation to the next bead from you, and stare for 5 seconds.

7. When all the beads have been clear and single, one at a time, move your fixation back to the near bead, and move an inch closer. Repeat the process. Each time you return to the near bead, move it another inch closer until it touches your nose.

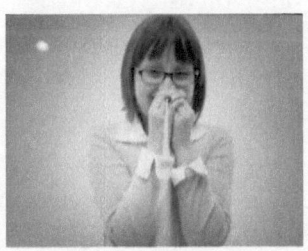

Example of Brock String

BI Stereograms:

1. Download an app for a tablet, or search google images for Stereograms. You may also get books with Stereograms from the library or book store. You will want a piece of glass or clear lucite to place over the Stereograms images if the page/screen is not reflective. An iPad is perfect with the shiny screen.

2. With the image of the Stereograms on the screen, set it approximately 12-16 inches away from you.

3. Hold a flashlight (penlight) next to you ear, aimed at the screen where the Stereograms is.

4. When looking at the Stereograms picture, you will see two flashlight images on the screen. When looking at the image of the flashlight, in order to make the flashlight appear as one, you will need to look as if you are looking through the screen. It will feel like looking out a window.

5. While staring at the image of the flashlight, the Stereogram picture will be blurry. Keep looking at the flashlight only, you will notice the stereogram in your peripheral (side) vision. All of a sudden, a three dimensional picture will jump out at you. This takes a lot of patience, and is a very difficult exercise to perform. When the image appears, don't try to look back at the picture to see it. The only way you will be able to see the 3D is to look through the page.

6.   Once you hold the image for a few minutes, you can try to move the flashlight away and hold the three dimensional image.

BO Stereograms:

1. Download an app for a tablet, or search google images for Stereograms. You may also get books with Stereograms from the library or book store. You will want a piece of glass or clear lucite to place over the Stereograms images if the image is not reflective. An Ipad is perfect with the shiny screen.

2. With the image of the Stereograms on the screen, set it approximately 12-16 inches away from you.

3. Hold a pointer, pencil, pen, or other thin target directly between you and the screen. It should be exactly in between you and the tablet. So if the screen is 12" away, hold the pointer at 6".

4. Stare at the pointer. If your eyes are aligned at the pointer (which is what you want), you

will only see one. If your eyes are aligned at the stereogram, you will see two pointers.

5. While staring at the pointer the stereogram behind it will become blurry. Keep looking at the pointer only.

6. All of a sudden, a three dimensional picture will jump out at you. This takes a lot of patience, and is a very difficult exercise to perform. When the image appears, don't try to look back at the picture to see it. The only way you will be able to see the 3D is to look at the pointer above the page. The picture will look like a footprint, pushed into the screen when you do this exercise.

Example of Stereograms

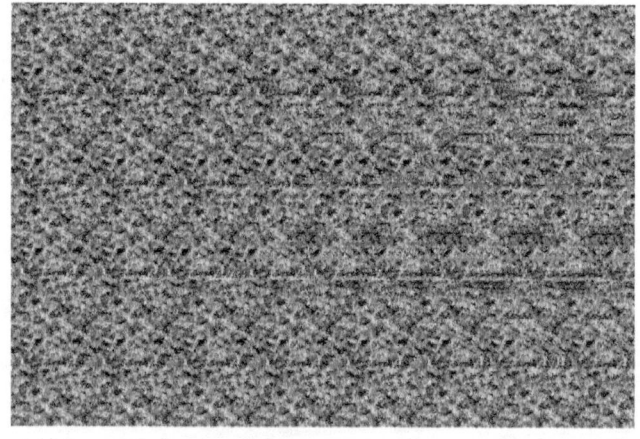

Definitions

Accommodative Esotropia – or refractive esotropia, is one of the most common forms of crossed eyes. It refers to eye crossing that is caused by the focusing efforts of the eyes as they try to see clearly. These patients are usually farsighted (or Hyperopic).

Accommodation – the ability to change focus of the eye from distance to near is a process achieved by the lens changing shape inside the eye.

Anterior segment of the eye – the cavity in the front third of the eye that includes the cornea, iris, cilliary body, aqueous humor, and lens.

Astigmatism – the imperfection of the curvature of the cornea, or in the shape of the eyes natural lens. This will cause multiple focus points of the light entering the eye.

Attention Deficit Disorder – any of a range of behavioral disorders occurring primarily in children, including such symptoms of poor concentration, hyperactivity, and impulsivity.

Attention Deficit Hyperactivity Disorder – when a person is unable to control behavior due to difficulty in processing neural stimuli, followed by a high level of motor activity.

Convergence Insufficiency – difficulty turning both eyes inward towards the nose when viewing near objects.

Cornea – transparent layer of tissue forming the front surface of the eye.

Dyslexia – a general term for disorders that involve difficulty in learning to read or interpret words, letters, and other symbols, but does not affect general intelligence.

Esotropia – a form of strabismus in which one or both of the eyes turn inward towards the nose. Also known as crossed eyes.

Exotropia – a form of strabismus where the eyes are deviated outward from the nose. The opposite of Esotropia.

Farsighted – unable to see things clearly, especially if they are relatively close to the eyes. The eye is structurally smaller than the focusing of light transmitting through the eye, causing the light rays to focus behind the eye. Also called Hyperopic.

Functional Eye Problem – the difficulty coordinating the many aspects involved in vision and visual processing. This is a problem that is usually not anatomical, and can usually be retrained.

Global Search Mechanism – ability to notice and identify words by the shape when not looking directly at them. Using peripheral vision mainly, one can read complete chunks of information without making the eye looks directly at each word.

Harmon's Distance – considered the optimal visual distance for reading and other close work. It is measured by finding the distance from your knuckles to your elbow of the same arm.

Iris – a flat colored ring shaped membrane behind the cornea of the eye, with an adjustable circular opening (pupil) in the center. It's main function is to control the amount of light entering the eye.

Learning Disability – a condition giving rise to difficulties in acquiring knowledge and skills, not associated with a physical handicap. They might have difficulty with reading, writing, spelling, reasoning, recalling, and organizing information.

Masking – hide, conceal, or disguise. In vision, masking is erasing the image interpreted by the retina, so a new image may be seen.

Nearsighted – unable to see things clearly unless they are relatively close to the eyes. The eye is structurally longer than the focus point of light, which creates the rays of light focusing in front of the retina. Also named Myopia.

Occipital Cortex – one of the four main lobes of the cerebral cortex of the brain. The occipital lobe is the visual processing center of the brain.

Optic Nerve – a nerve that connects the eye to the brain. Carries impulses from the retina which can be interpreted in the brain to give sight.

Perception – the organization, identification, and interpretation of sensory information in order to represent and understand information presented.

Posterior Segment Of The Eye – the cavity of the back two thirds of the eye that includes the vitreous humor, retina, choroid, and optic nerve.

Pursuit Eye Movements – the smooth movement, allowing the eyes to closely track or follow a moving object.

Refractive Amblyopia – when there is a large or unequal amount of refractive error (glasses strength) between the two eyes. The brain chooses one eye to be the dominant eye, and the other may not develop fully.

Retina – the layer lining the back of the eye contains cells that are sensitive to light, and trigger nerve impulses that pass via the optic nerve to the brain to create a visual image.

Saccadic Eye Movement – a quick movement of both eyes between fixation points.

Stereopsis – the perception of depth produced by the brain receiving information from both eyes.

Strabismus – the abnormal alignment of the eyes.